DIABETIC RECIPES FOR NEWLY DIAGNOSED

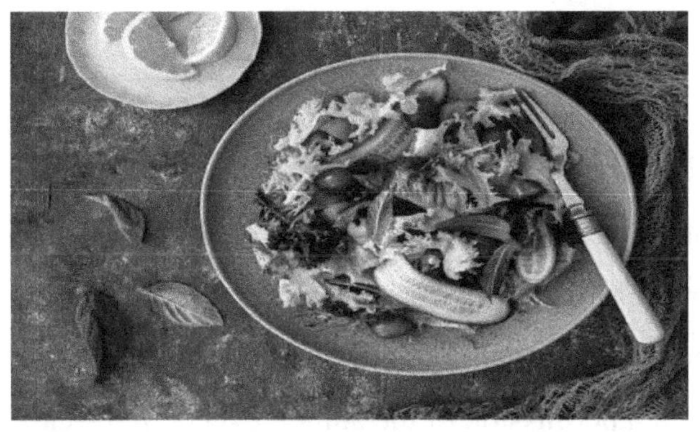

Your Journey To An Overall
Well-being

Karla Mayer

TABLE OF CONTENTS

INTRODUCTION

"Diabetic Recipes for Newly Diagnosed," is a comprehensive guide designed to support individuals who are navigating life with diabetes for the first time. Being diagnosed with diabetes can be overwhelming, but it doesn't mean sacrificing flavor or enjoyment in your meals. In fact, it's an opportunity to embrace a healthier lifestyle through mindful eating and delicious, nutritious recipes tailored to your needs.

This book is crafted with care and expertise, drawing upon the latest research in diabetes management and culinary innovation to provide you with practical solutions and mouth watering dishes. Whether you're seeking guidance on meal planning, looking for tasty alternatives to your favorite foods, or simply in need of support and encouragement, you'll find everything you need within these pages.

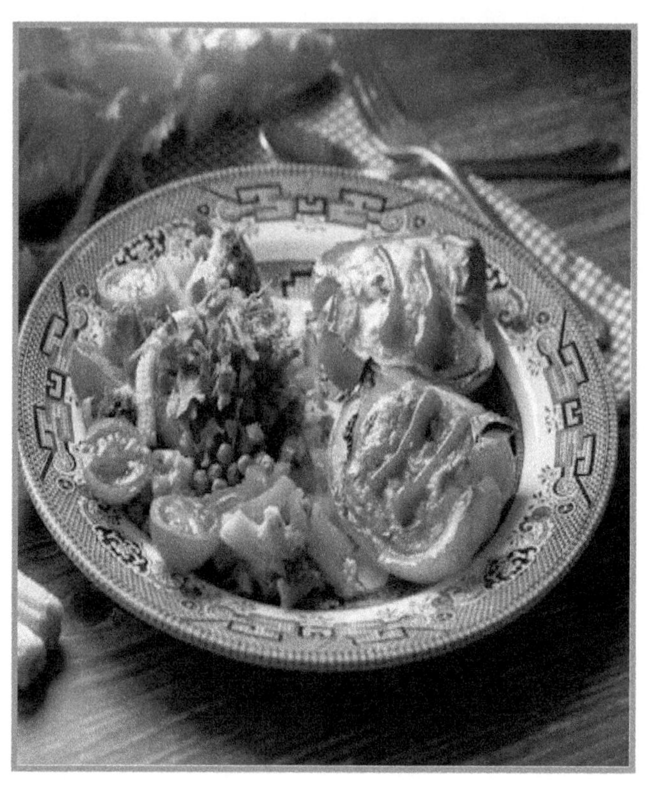

CHAPTER ONE

Understanding Diabetes

Upon receiving a diabetes diagnosis, understanding the condition becomes paramount. In this chapter, we'll delve into the basics of diabetes, including its types, causes, symptoms, and how it affects your body. Armed with this knowledge, you'll be better equipped to navigate your journey towards optimal health and well-being.

Diabetes is a chronic condition characterized by elevated blood sugar levels resulting from either insufficient insulin production or the body's inability to effectively use insulin. Type 1, type 2, and gestational diabetes are the three main forms of the disease..

When the immune system unintentionally targets and kills the pancreatic beta cells that produce insulin, type 1 diabetes results.. This leads to a lack of insulin, requiring daily insulin injections for survival. Type 1 diabetes can strike at any age, but it usually appears in childhood or adolescence.

Type 2 diabetes, on the other hand, develops when the body becomes resistant to insulin or fails to produce enough insulin to maintain normal blood sugar levels. This type of diabetes is more common and is often associated with lifestyle factors such as poor diet, lack of exercise, and obesity. While type 2 diabetes can occur at any age, it is more prevalent in adults.

Gestational diabetes occurs during pregnancy when the body cannot produce enough insulin to meet the increased demand. While it usually resolves after childbirth, women who have had gestational diabetes are at higher risk of developing type 2 diabetes later in life.

Regardless of the type, diabetes can have serious complications if left unmanaged. These include cardiovascular disease, nerve damage, kidney damage, and vision loss. However, with proper treatment and lifestyle modifications, many of these complications can be prevented or delayed.

Increased thirst, frequent urination, unexplained weight loss, exhaustion, hazy eyesight, and sluggish wound healing are some signs of diabetes. However, some people may have diabetes without experiencing any symptoms, which is why regular screening and monitoring are essential, especially for those at higher risk.

Understanding the basics of diabetes is the first step towards effectively managing the condition. By taking an active role in your health and making informed choices, you can live a full and fulfilling life with diabetes. In the following chapters, we'll explore practical strategies and delicious recipes to help you on your journey to better health and well-being.

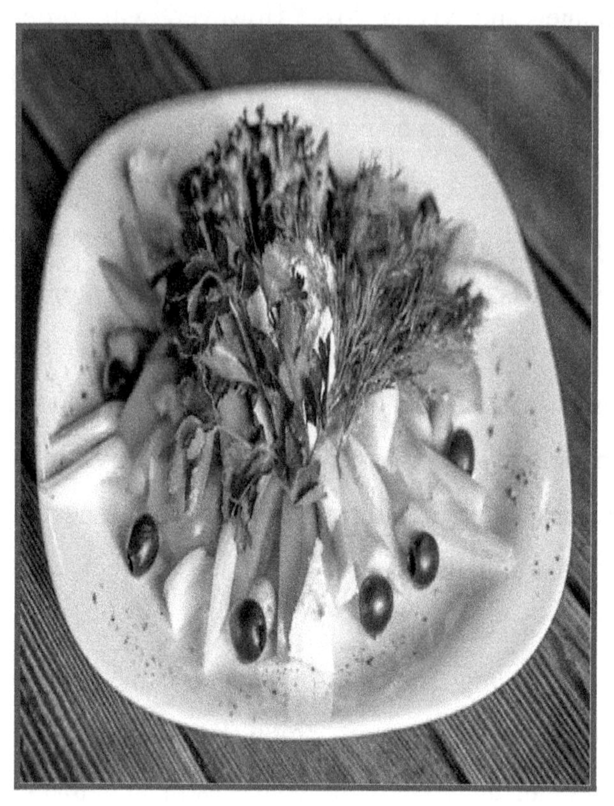

CHAPTER TWO

The Importance of Nutrition in Managing Diabetes

Nutrition plays a fundamental role in managing diabetes effectively. What you eat directly impacts your blood sugar levels, making it crucial to adopt a balanced and mindful approach to your diet. In this chapter, we'll explore the significance of nutrition in diabetes management, learn about key nutrients, and discover how to create delicious, diabetes-friendly meals that promote stable blood sugar levels and overall well-being.

Understanding Carbohydrates

Carbohydrates have the most significant impact on blood sugar levels, making them a focal point in diabetes meal planning. When consumed, carbohydrates are broken down into glucose, raising blood sugar levels. However, not all carbohydrates are created equal. Understanding the concept of glycemic index (GI) and glycemic load (GL) can help you make informed choices.

Low GI foods take longer to digest and absorb, which causes blood sugar levels to rise gradually. These include whole grains, legumes, non-starchy vegetables, and fruits such as berries and apples. On the other hand, foods with a high GI, such as white bread, white rice, and sugary snacks, cause a rapid spike in blood sugar levels and should be consumed in moderation.

Balancing Macronutrients

In addition to carbohydrates, it's essential to consider protein and fat in your meals. Protein helps stabilize blood sugar levels and promotes feelings of fullness, while healthy fats provide sustained energy and support overall health. Aim to include lean sources of protein, such as poultry, fish, tofu, and legumes, in each meal. Incorporate healthy fats from sources like avocados, nuts, seeds, and olive oil to add flavor and satiety.

Fiber-Rich Foods

Fiber is beneficial for people with diabetes as it helps slow down the absorption of sugar and improves blood sugar control. It also aids in digestion, promotes heart health, and contributes to weight management. Focus on incorporating fiber-rich foods into your diet, including whole grains, fruits, vegetables, nuts, seeds, and legumes. Aim for a variety of colors and textures to maximize nutritional benefits.

Portion Control and Mindful Eating

Managing portion sizes is key to controlling blood sugar levels and preventing overeating. Pay attention to serving sizes and practice mindful eating by listening to your body's hunger and fullness cues. When dining, stay away from distractions like watching TV or browsing through your phone and take time to enjoy every bite. Eating slowly allows your brain to register feelings of satisfaction, reducing the likelihood of overeating.

Meal Planning Strategies

Effective meal planning is essential for maintaining stable blood sugar levels and achieving nutritional goals. Start by creating a weekly meal plan that includes a variety of nutrient-rich foods from all food groups. Incorporate a balance of carbohydrates, protein, and fats into each meal and snack to promote satiety and prevent blood sugar spikes.

Consider prepping meals and snacks in advance to save time and ensure healthy options are readily available. Stock your kitchen with diabetes-friendly ingredients, such as whole grains, lean proteins, fresh fruits and vegetables, and healthy fats. Try varying the flavors and cooking techniques to make your meals interesting and pleasurable.

Diabetes-Friendly Recipes

Now that we've covered the basics of nutrition in diabetes management, let's explore some delicious recipes tailored to support stable blood sugar levels and overall health. From hearty salads and flavorful stir-fries to satisfying soups and comforting casseroles, there are endless possibilities for creating nutritious and delicious meals that you'll love to eat.

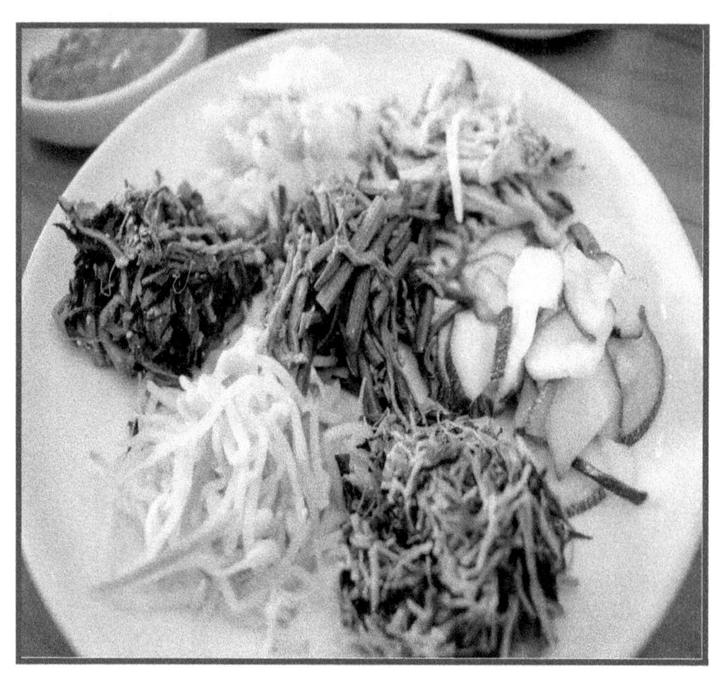

CHAPTER THREE

Wholesome Breakfasts to Start Your Day Off Right

For good reason, breakfast is frequently heralded as the most significant meal of the day.. For individuals managing diabetes, starting the day with a balanced and nutritious breakfast can set the tone for stable blood sugar levels and overall well-being. In this chapter, we will explore a variety of wholesome breakfast options tailored to meet the needs of those newly diagnosed with diabetes. From whole grain choices to protein-rich dishes, fruit and vegetable options, and low-carb alternatives, we have curated a selection of recipes to inspire your mornings and help you kickstart your day on a healthy note.

Whole Grain Options

Whole grains are a fantastic source of fiber and nutrients, making them an excellent choice for individuals with diabetes. They help regulate blood sugar levels and provide sustained energy throughout the morning. Here are some delicious whole grain breakfast options to try:

Steel-Cut Oats with Berries and Nuts

Start your day with a warm bowl of steel-cut oats topped with a colorful mix of berries and a sprinkle of nuts for added crunch and protein.

Avocado Toast on Whole Grain Bread

Mash ripe avocado onto a slice of whole grain bread and top with a drizzle of olive oil, a sprinkle of sea salt, and a dash of red pepper flakes for a satisfying and nutritious breakfast.

Brown Rice Pudding with Cinnamon and Raisins

Transform leftover brown rice into a creamy and comforting pudding by simmering it with almond milk, cinnamon, and sweet raisins for a hearty morning treat.

Protein-Rich Options

Protein plays a crucial role in managing blood sugar levels and keeping you feeling full and satisfied. Incorporating protein-rich foods into your breakfast can help stabilize your energy levels throughout the day. Here are some protein-packed breakfast ideas:

Scrambled Tofu with Veggies and Salsa
Swap out traditional scrambled eggs for tofu seasoned with your favorite veggies and a dollop of zesty salsa for a flavorful and plant-based breakfast.
Greek Yogurt Parfait with Granola and Fruit
Layer creamy Greek yogurt with crunchy granola and a medley of fresh fruits for a refreshing and protein-rich parfait that is as delicious as it is nutritious.

Spinach and Feta Omelette
Whip up a fluffy omelette filled with sautéed spinach and crumbled feta cheese for a savory and protein-packed breakfast that will keep you satisfied until lunchtime.

Fruit and Vegetable Options

Incorporating fruits and vegetables into your breakfast not only adds a burst of flavor and color but also provides essential vitamins and minerals to support your overall health. Here are some vibrant fruit and vegetable breakfast ideas to try:

Green Smoothie with Kale, Spinach, and Apple
Blend together a handful of leafy greens, a crisp apple, and a splash of coconut water for a refreshing and nutrient-packed green smoothie to kickstart your day.

Berry and Chia Seed Smoothie Bowl
Top a thick and creamy berry smoothie with a sprinkle of chia seeds, fresh berries, and a drizzle of honey for a satisfying and antioxidant-rich breakfast bowl.

Roasted Vegetable and Feta Frittata
Bake a colorful frittata filled with roasted vegetables and tangy feta cheese for a hearty and

veggie-packed breakfast that is perfect for sharing with family and friends.

Low-Carb Options

For individuals looking to manage their carbohydrate intake, low-carb breakfast options can be a great choice. These recipes are designed to be satisfying and delicious while keeping your blood sugar levels in check. Here are some low-carb breakfast ideas to explore:

Chia Seed Pudding with Almond Milk and Berries
Mix chia seeds with almond milk and a handful of fresh berries for a creamy and low-carb pudding that is rich in fiber and omega-3 fatty acids.

Spinach and Cheese Egg Muffins
Bake individual egg muffins loaded with spinach, cheese, and herbs for a convenient and protein-packed breakfast that can be enjoyed on the go.

Coconut Milk Yogurt with Nuts and Seeds

Enjoy a bowl of dairy-free coconut milk yogurt topped with a mix of crunchy nuts, seeds, and a drizzle of honey for a satisfying and low-carb breakfast option that is both creamy and nutritious.

In a nutshell, breakfast is a wonderful opportunity to nourish your body and set a positive tone for the day ahead. By incorporating a variety of wholesome and delicious breakfast options into your routine, you can support your overall health and well-being while managing your diabetes effectively. Experiment with these recipes, get creative in the kitchen, and discover what works best for you. Remember, breakfast is not just a meal; it's a chance to care for yourself and start each day with intention and vitality. Here's to many more delicious and nutritious breakfasts on your journey to wellness.

CHAPTER FOUR

Delicious Lunch Ideas for Diabetics

Lunch is an essential part of your daily routine, providing you with the energy and nutrients you need to power through the rest of the day. For individuals managing diabetes, choosing the right lunch options can help support stable blood sugar levels and overall well-being. In this chapter, we will explore a variety of nourishing lunch options tailored to meet the needs of those newly diagnosed with diabetes. From leafy green salads to hearty soups and stews, sandwiches and wraps, and grain bowls and salads, we have curated a selection of recipes to inspire your midday meals and help you enjoy delicious and healthy lunches.

Leafy Green Salads

Leafy greens are a fantastic source of fiber, vitamins, and minerals, making them an excellent choice for individuals with diabetes. They are low in calories and carbohydrates, yet high in nutrients that support overall health. Here are some delicious leafy green salad options to try:

Kale and Quinoa Salad with Roasted Vegetables and Lemon-Tahini Dressing

Massage kale with a drizzle of olive oil and mix with cooked quinoa, roasted vegetables, and a tangy lemon-tahini dressing for a hearty and nutritious salad.

Spinach and Strawberry Salad with Goat Cheese and Balsamic Glaze

Toss fresh spinach with sliced strawberries, crumbled goat cheese, and a sweet balsamic glaze for a refreshing and flavorful salad that is perfect for summer.

Arugula and Beet Salad with Avocado and Citrus Vinaigrette

Combine peppery arugula with roasted beets, creamy avocado, and a zesty citrus vinaigrette for a colorful and nutrient-packed salad that is both beautiful and delicious.

Hearty Soups and Stews

Soups and stews are a great way to incorporate a variety of nutrients and flavors into your lunch. They are also an excellent option for those who prefer a warm and comforting meal during colder months. Here are some hearty soup and stew options to try:

Lentil Soup with Tomatoes, Carrots, and Kale
Simmer lentils with diced tomatoes, carrots, and kale for a filling and fiber-rich soup that is both satisfying and nutritious.

Chicken and Vegetable Stew with Quinoa and Herbs
Slow cook chicken and a variety of vegetables with quinoa and herbs for a flavorful and protein-packed stew that will keep you full and energized throughout the afternoon.

Minestrone Soup with White Beans, Zucchini, and Pasta

Combine white beans, zucchini, pasta, and a medley of vegetables in a flavorful broth for a comforting and hearty soup that is perfect for a quick and easy lunch.

Sandwiches and Wraps

Sandwiches and wraps are a convenient and versatile lunch option that can be customized to meet your individual needs and preferences. Here are some healthy sandwich and wrap options to try:

Turkey and Avocado Wrap with Whole Grain Tortilla and Sprouts

Roll sliced turkey, avocado, lettuce, tomato, and sprouts in a whole grain tortilla for a satisfying and protein-packed wrap that is both delicious and nutritious.

Hummus and Veggie Sandwich with Whole Grain Bread and Pesto

Spread hummus on whole grain bread and top with your favorite vegetables, such as lettuce, tomato, cucumber, and red onion, for a refreshing and flavorful sandwich that is high in fiber and protein.

Grilled Chicken and Pesto Panini with Whole Grain Bread and Roasted Vegetables

Grill a chicken and pesto panini with roasted vegetables, such as zucchini, bell peppers, and onions, for a savory and satisfying lunch that is both delicious and filling.

Grain Bowls and Salads

Grain bowls and salads are a great way to incorporate a variety of nutrients and flavors into your lunch. They are also a convenient and portable option for those who are on-the-go. Here are some healthy grain bowl and salad options to try:

Quinoa and Black Bean Bowl topped with lime, avocado, and salsa

Combine cooked quinoa with black beans, diced avocado, salsa, and a squeeze of lime for a filling and fiber-rich bowl that is both satisfying and nutritious.

Buddha Bowl with Roasted Vegetables, Tofu, and Peanut Sauce

Fill a bowl with roasted vegetables, tofu, and your favorite grains, such as brown rice or quinoa, and top with a flavorful peanut sauce for a plant-based and protein-packed lunch.

Chicken and Vegetable Grain Salad with Lemon-Tahini Dressing

Mix cooked grains, such as farro or barley, with cooked chicken, roasted vegetables, and a tangy lemon-tahini dressing for a hearty and nutritious salad that is perfect for a quick and easy lunch.

Lunch is an important part of your daily routine, providing you with the energy and nutrients you need to power through the rest of the day. By incorporating a variety of nourishing and delicious lunch options into your routine, you can support your overall health and well-being while managing your diabetes effectively. Experiment with these recipes, get creative in the kitchen, and discover what works best for you. Remember, lunch is not just a meal; it's a chance to care for yourself and enjoy a delicious and nutritious midday break. Here's to many more nourishing and satisfying lunches on your journey to wellness!

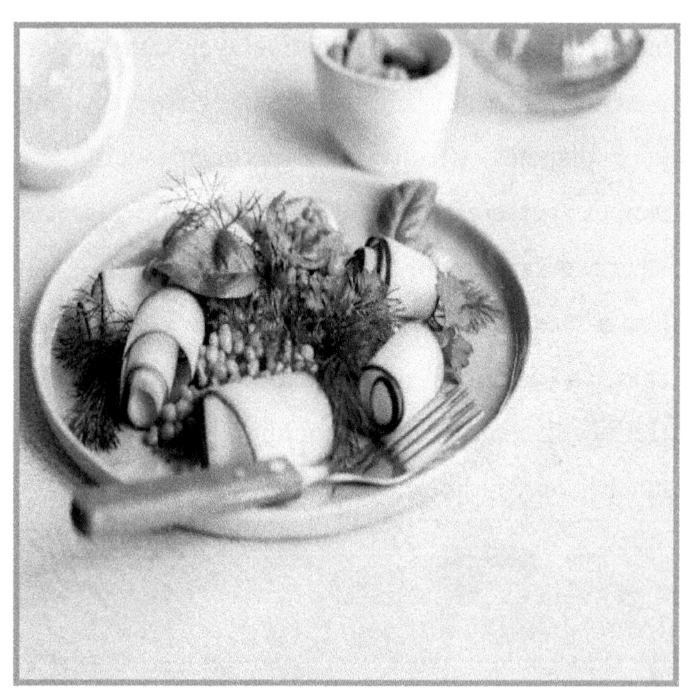

CHAPTER FIVE

Nourishing Dinner Recipes to Support Diabetes Management

As the day winds down, dinner presents an opportunity to unwind and nourish your body with a satisfying meal. For individuals managing diabetes, dinner is a critical time to focus on nutrient-dense foods that help maintain stable blood sugar levels while satisfying your taste buds. In this chapter, we'll explore a variety of nourishing dinner recipes designed to support diabetes management, promote overall health, and bring joy to your table.

Baked Salmon with Roasted Vegetables:

Start your evening with a heart-healthy meal featuring baked salmon and roasted vegetables. Season salmon fillets with olive oil, lemon juice, minced garlic, and fresh herbs such as dill or parsley. Place the salmon on a baking sheet lined with parchment paper and surround it with a medley of colorful vegetables such as broccoli, bell peppers, carrots, and Brussels sprouts. Drizzle the vegetables with olive oil, season with salt and pepper, and roast in the oven until tender and caramelized. Serve the baked salmon alongside the roasted vegetables for a balanced and flavorful dinner option.

Turkey and Vegetable Stir-Fry:

Whip up a quick and delicious turkey and vegetable stir-fry for a satisfying dinner that's bursting with flavor. Begin by sautéing lean ground turkey in a hot skillet with minced garlic, grated ginger, and a splash of low-sodium soy sauce or tamari. Once the turkey is cooked through, add a variety of colorful vegetables such as bell peppers, snap peas, broccoli, and carrots. Stir-fry until the vegetables are crisp-tender, then add a drizzle of sesame oil and sprinkle with sesame seeds for added crunch and flavor. Serve the turkey and vegetable stir-fry over cooked brown rice or cauliflower rice for a nutritious and filling meal.

Spaghetti Squash with Turkey Bolognese:

Swap traditional pasta for nutrient-rich spaghetti squash in this lighter take on classic spaghetti with Bolognese sauce. Begin by roasting a spaghetti squash in the oven until tender. Meanwhile, prepare a flavorful turkey Bolognese sauce by sautéing lean ground turkey with onions, garlic, diced tomatoes, tomato paste, and Italian herbs. Simmer the sauce until thick and fragrant, then toss it with the cooked spaghetti squash strands. Top with a sprinkle of grated Parmesan cheese and fresh basil for a satisfying and comforting dinner option that's low in carbs and high in flavor.

Chickpea and Vegetable Curry:

Warm up with a cozy and aromatic chickpea and vegetable curry that's packed with protein and fiber. Begin by sautéing diced onions, garlic, and ginger in a large pot until fragrant. Add your favorite curry spices such as turmeric, cumin, coriander, and garam masala, and toast them briefly to release their flavors. Stir in diced vegetables such as cauliflower, bell peppers, and sweet potatoes, along with canned chickpeas and coconut milk.Once the flavors have combined and the vegetables are soft, simmer the curry. Serve the chickpea and vegetable curry over cooked brown rice or quinoa for a nourishing and satisfying dinner option.

Stuffed Bell Peppers with Quinoa and Black Beans

Enjoy a wholesome and colorful dinner with stuffed bell peppers filled with a hearty mixture of quinoa, black beans, vegetables, and spices. Begin by halving bell peppers and removing the seeds and membranes. Cook quinoa according to package instructions and mix it with black beans, diced tomatoes, corn kernels, diced onions, and minced garlic. Season with chili powder, cumin, and smoked paprika for added flavor. Stuff the quinoa and black bean mixture into the bell pepper halves and bake in the oven until the peppers are tender and the filling is heated through. Top with a dollop of Greek yogurt and chopped cilantro for a fresh and flavorful dinner option.

Grilled Chicken with Greek Salad:

Transport your taste buds to the Mediterranean with a light and refreshing Greek salad paired with grilled chicken. Marinate chicken breasts in lemon juice, olive oil, minced garlic, and dried oregano for added flavor. Grill the chicken until cooked through and lightly charred, then slice it thinly. Toss together a Greek salad with diced cucumbers, cherry tomatoes, red onions, Kalamata olives, and crumbled feta cheese. Dress the salad with a simple vinaigrette made with olive oil, red wine vinegar, and dried oregano. Serve the grilled chicken alongside the Greek salad for a satisfying and nutritious dinner option that's bursting with Mediterranean flavors.

Vegetable and Lentil Soup:

Cozy up with a comforting bowl of vegetable and lentil soup that's perfect for chilly evenings. Begin by sautéing diced onions, carrots, and celery in olive oil until softened. Add dried lentils, vegetable broth, diced tomatoes, and your favorite herbs and spices such as thyme, rosemary, and bay leaves. Simmer the soup until the lentils are tender and the vegetables are cooked through. Stir in chopped kale or spinach for added nutrition and freshness. Serve the vegetable and lentil soup hot with a slice of whole-grain bread or a side of crackers for a satisfying and nourishing dinner option.

Baked Chicken Parmesan with Zucchini Noodles:

Indulge in a lighter take on classic chicken Parmesan with baked chicken breasts served over zucchini noodles. Begin by coating chicken breasts in a mixture of whole-wheat breadcrumbs, grated Parmesan cheese, and Italian herbs. Bake the chicken until it's cooked through and golden brown.Meanwhile, spiralize zucchini into noodles and sauté them in olive oil until tender. Top the zucchini noodles with marinara sauce and place a baked chicken breast on top. Sprinkle with additional Parmesan cheese and fresh basil for a healthier twist on a beloved Italian dish.

Tofu and Vegetable Curry with Cauliflower Rice:

Enjoy a plant-based dinner option with tofu and vegetable curry served over cauliflower rice. Begin by pressing tofu to remove excess moisture, then cut it into cubes. Sauté the tofu in a hot skillet with diced onions, bell peppers, and zucchini until golden brown. Add your favorite curry paste or powder along with canned coconut milk and simmer until the vegetables are tender and the flavors have melded together. Serve the tofu and vegetable curry over cooked cauliflower rice for a low-carb alternative to traditional rice. Garnish with chopped cilantro and a squeeze of lime juice for a burst of freshness.

Shrimp and Vegetable Stir-Fry with Brown Rice:
Whip up a quick and flavorful shrimp and vegetable stir-fry for a nutritious and satisfying dinner option. Begin by sautéing shrimp in a hot skillet with minced garlic, grated ginger, and a splash of low-sodium soy sauce or tamari. Once the shrimp is cooked through, remove it from the skillet and set it aside. In the same skillet, stir-fry a mix of colorful vegetables such as bell peppers, snap peas, broccoli, and carrots until crisp-tender. Add cooked shrimp back to the skillet and toss with your favorite stir-fry sauce. Serve the shrimp and vegetable stir-fry over cooked brown rice for a balanced and delicious meal.

Dinner is a time to unwind, nourish your body, and enjoy the company of loved ones. With these nourishing dinner recipes tailored to support diabetes management, you can savor delicious meals while maintaining stable blood sugar levels and promoting overall health. From flavorful grilled chicken salads to comforting lentil soups and vibrant vegetable stir-fries, there's something for everyone to enjoy. Experiment with different ingredients, flavors, and cooking techniques to keep your dinners exciting and satisfying. With a little creativity and planning, you can indulge in nutritious and delicious meals that support your well-being, one bite at a time.

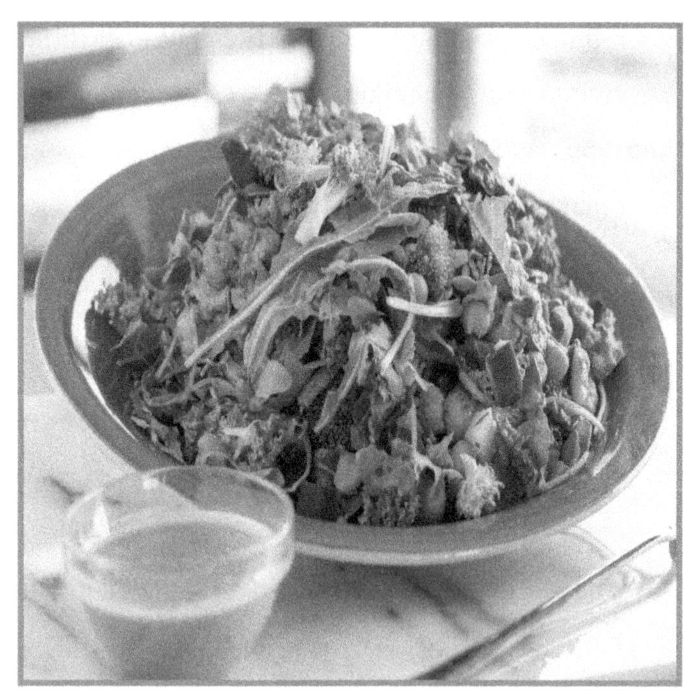

CHAPTER SIX

Snack Time: Healthy Options for Diabetic Diets

Snacking can be a crucial part of managing diabetes, helping to keep blood sugar levels stable between meals and preventing overeating later in the day. However, it's essential to choose snacks that are nutritious, satisfying, and low in added sugars and refined carbohydrates. In this chapter, we'll explore a variety of healthy snack options specifically tailored to support diabetic diets, providing both delicious flavors and essential nutrients to keep you feeling energized and satisfied throughout the day.

Fresh Fruit with Nut Butter:
Pairing fresh fruit with nut butter is a simple and satisfying snack option that combines natural sweetness with healthy fats and protein. Choose fruits with a lower glycemic index, such as berries,

apples, or pear slices, and pair them with a tablespoon of almond butter, peanut butter, or cashew butter. The fiber and protein in the nut butter help slow down the absorption of sugar from the fruit, providing a steady source of energy and keeping you feeling full and satisfied until your next meal.

Greek Yogurt with Berries and Nuts:

Greek yogurt is a protein-rich snack that can help stabilize blood sugar levels and promote feelings of fullness. Top a serving of plain Greek yogurt with a handful of fresh berries, such as strawberries, blueberries, or raspberries, for natural sweetness and a boost of antioxidants. Sprinkle with a tablespoon of chopped nuts, such as almonds, walnuts, or pecans, for added crunch and healthy fats. This combination provides a balanced mix of protein, fiber, and healthy carbohydrates to keep you satisfied and energized throughout the day.

Veggie Sticks with Hummus:

Crunchy vegetable sticks paired with creamy hummus make for a satisfying and nutritious snack that's packed with fiber, vitamins, and minerals. Cut up raw vegetables such as carrots, celery, cucumber, and bell peppers into sticks or slices for easy dipping. Pair with a serving of hummus made from chickpeas, tahini, lemon juice, and garlic for added protein and flavor. The combination of crunchy veggies and creamy hummus provides a satisfying snack that's low in calories and high in nutrition, making it perfect for managing diabetes.

Hard-Boiled Eggs with Whole-Grain Crackers:

Hard-boiled eggs are a convenient and portable snack option that's rich in protein and essential nutrients. Pair a hard-boiled egg with a serving of whole-grain crackers for a balanced snack that provides both protein and complex carbohydrates. The combination of protein and fiber helps keep blood sugar levels stable and promotes feelings of fullness and satiety. Packaged in individual containers, hard-boiled eggs and whole-grain crackers make a perfect on-the-go snack option for busy days.

Cottage Cheese with Tomato Slices and Basil:
Cottage cheese is a protein-packed snack that's low in carbohydrates and provides essential nutrients such as calcium and phosphorus. Top a serving of cottage cheese with slices of fresh tomato and a few basil leaves for a refreshing and flavorful snack option. The combination of creamy cottage cheese, juicy tomato slices, and fragrant basil creates a delicious and satisfying snack that's perfect for any time of day. Enjoy it as a mid-morning pick-me-up or a light afternoon snack to keep you feeling full and energized.

Trail Mix with Nuts, Seeds, and Dried Fruit:
Trail mix is a convenient and customizable snack option that's perfect for managing diabetes. Make your own trail mix by combining a variety of nuts,

seeds, and dried fruit for a balanced mix of protein, healthy fats, and carbohydrates. Choose unsalted nuts such as almonds, walnuts, and cashews, along with seeds like pumpkin seeds and sunflower seeds. Add in a small amount of dried fruit such as raisins, cranberries, or apricots for natural sweetness and extra flavor. Portion out individual servings of trail mix into small containers or snack bags for easy grab-and-go snacking throughout the day.

Avocado Toast on Whole-Grain Bread:

Avocado toast is a delicious and nutritious snack option that's packed with heart-healthy fats and fiber. Mash half an avocado onto a slice of whole-grain bread and sprinkle with a pinch of salt and pepper. For extra flavor and nutrition, add toppings such as sliced tomatoes, cucumber slices, or a sprinkle of red pepper flakes. The combination of creamy avocado and hearty whole-grain bread provides a satisfying snack that's perfect for any time of day. Enjoy it as a quick and easy breakfast, a mid-morning snack, or a light afternoon pick-me-up to keep you feeling full and satisfied.

Edamame with Sea Salt:

Edamame, or young soybeans, are a nutrient-rich snack that's packed with protein, fiber, and essential vitamins and minerals. Simply steam or boil edamame pods until tender, then sprinkle with a pinch of sea salt for added flavor. Edamame makes a satisfying and nutritious snack that's perfect for managing diabetes. Enjoy it as a standalone snack or incorporate it into salads, stir-fries, or grain bowls for added protein and texture.

Tuna Salad Lettuce Wraps:

Tuna salad lettuce wraps are a light and refreshing snack option that's perfect for managing diabetes. Mix canned tuna with Greek yogurt, diced celery, red onion, and a squeeze of lemon juice for added flavor. Spoon the tuna salad onto large lettuce leaves, such as romaine or butter lettuce, and roll them up like wraps. The combination of protein-rich tuna and crisp lettuce leaves provides a satisfying snack that's low in carbohydrates and perfect for any time of day.

Dark Chocolate-Covered Almonds:

Indulge your sweet tooth with dark chocolate-covered almonds, a delicious and satisfying snack option that's perfect for managing diabetes. Choose dark chocolate with a high cocoa content for maximum health benefits and minimal added sugars. Dip whole almonds into melted dark chocolate and place them on a parchment-lined baking sheet to set. Once the chocolate has hardened, enjoy these decadent treats as a guilt-free snack that's rich in antioxidants, fiber, and healthy fats.

Incorporating these healthy snack options into your daily routine can help you manage diabetes effectively while satisfying your cravings and keeping you feeling energized and satisfied throughout the day. Experiment with different flavors, textures, and combinations to find your favorite snacks that support your health and well-being. Whether you prefer sweet or savory, crunchy or creamy, there's a healthy snack option for everyone to enjoy on their journey to better health with diabetes.

CHAPTER SEVEN

Decadent Desserts without the Blood Sugar Spike

Desserts are often viewed as off-limits for individuals managing diabetes, but it doesn't have to be that way. With the right ingredients and recipes, you can indulge in decadent desserts that satisfy your sweet tooth without causing a blood sugar spike. In this chapter, we'll explore a variety of delicious dessert options specifically tailored to support diabetes management, allowing you to enjoy a treat without compromising your health.

Flourless Chocolate Cake:

Sink your teeth into a rich and decadent flourless chocolate cake that's perfect for satisfying your chocolate cravings without the guilt. Made with almond flour, cocoa powder, eggs, and a touch of sweetness from maple syrup or stevia, this indulgent dessert is low in carbohydrates and high in flavor. Serve it with a dollop of whipped cream or a sprinkle of powdered sugar for an extra special treat that's sure to impress.

Berry Parfait with Greek Yogurt:

Layer fresh berries with creamy Greek yogurt and a sprinkle of granola for a delicious and nutritious parfait that's perfect for any time of day. Choose low-glycemic fruits such as strawberries, blueberries, and raspberries, which are packed with antioxidants and fiber. Greek yogurt adds a creamy texture and a boost of protein, while granola provides a satisfying crunch. Enjoy this guilt-free dessert as a refreshing snack or a light after-dinner treat that won't spike your blood sugar levels.

Avocado Chocolate Mousse:

Indulge in a creamy and decadent chocolate mousse made with avocado for a dessert that's both delicious and nutritious. Blend ripe avocados with cocoa powder, almond milk, and a natural sweetener such as honey or agave nectar until smooth and creamy. Chill the mousse in the refrigerator until set, then serve it topped with fresh berries or a sprinkle of chopped nuts for added flavor and texture. This luscious dessert is rich in healthy fats and antioxidants, making it a guilt-free treat for satisfying your chocolate cravings.

Coconut Flour Banana Bread:

Enjoy a slice of moist and flavorful banana bread made with coconut flour for a delicious and satisfying dessert option that's perfect for managing diabetes. Coconut flour is lower in carbohydrates and higher in fiber than traditional flour, making it a healthier choice for individuals watching their blood sugar levels. Sweetened with ripe bananas and a touch of honey or maple syrup, this banana bread is bursting with flavor and natural sweetness. Enjoy it warm from the oven with a smear of almond butter or cream cheese for an extra indulgent treat.

Chia Seed Pudding:

Treat yourself to a creamy and nutritious chia seed pudding that's packed with fiber, protein, and essential nutrients. Simply mix chia seeds with your favorite milk, such as almond milk or coconut milk, and a natural sweetener such as honey or stevia. Let the mixture sit in the refrigerator overnight to thicken, then serve it topped with fresh fruit, nuts, or shredded coconut for added flavor and texture. Chia seed pudding is a versatile dessert option that can be customized to suit your taste preferences and dietary needs, making it a perfect choice for individuals managing diabetes.

Baked Apples with Cinnamon and Walnuts:
Satisfy your sweet tooth with baked apples filled with cinnamon and walnuts for a comforting and nutritious dessert option that's perfect for cooler weather. Core apples and fill them with a mixture of chopped walnuts, cinnamon, and a touch of honey or maple syrup. Bake until the apples are tender and fragrant, then serve them warm with a scoop of Greek yogurt or a drizzle of caramel sauce for added indulgence. This simple yet satisfying dessert

is low in carbohydrates and high in fiber, making it a guilt-free treat for satisfying your sweet cravings.

Pumpkin Spice Energy Balls:
Whip up a batch of pumpkin spice energy balls for a tasty and nutritious dessert option that's perfect for on-the-go snacking. Made with pumpkin puree, oats, nut butter, and warm spices such as cinnamon, nutmeg, and ginger, these bite-sized treats are bursting with flavor and natural sweetness. Roll the mixture into balls and chill them in the refrigerator until firm, then enjoy them as a satisfying dessert or snack whenever you need a quick pick-me-up. Pumpkin spice energy balls are packed with fiber, protein, and healthy fats, making them a perfect choice for individuals managing diabetes.

Frozen Yogurt Bark with Berries and Almonds:
Cool off with a refreshing frozen yogurt bark topped with fresh berries and crunchy almonds for a delicious and nutritious dessert option that's perfect for hot summer days. Spread Greek yogurt onto a

baking sheet lined with parchment paper, then sprinkle with your favorite berries and chopped almonds. Freeze until firm, then break the bark into pieces and enjoy it as a guilt-free dessert or snack. Frozen yogurt bark is rich in protein, calcium, and antioxidants, making it a perfect choice for satisfying your sweet cravings while supporting your health.

Lemon Poppy Seed Muffins:

Indulge in a citrusy and fragrant lemon poppy seed muffin for a delicious and satisfying dessert option that's perfect for any time of day. Made with almond flour, Greek yogurt, and fresh lemon zest, these muffins are bursting with flavor and natural sweetness. Enjoy them warm from the oven with a cup of tea or coffee for a delightful treat that won't spike your blood sugar levels. Lemon poppy seed muffins are rich in protein, fiber, and essential nutrients, making them a perfect choice for individuals managing diabetes.

Chocolate-Dipped Strawberries:

Satisfy your chocolate cravings with chocolate-dipped strawberries for a simple and elegant dessert option that's perfect for special occasions or everyday indulgence. Dip fresh strawberries into melted dark chocolate and place them on a parchment-lined baking sheet to set. Once the chocolate has hardened, enjoy these sweet and juicy treats as a guilt-free dessert that's rich in antioxidants and fiber. Chocolate-dipped strawberries are a delicious and nutritious way to satisfy your sweet tooth while supporting your health and well-being.

You may efficiently manage your diabetes, indulge your sweet tooth, and improve your general health and well-being by including these rich desserts in your meal plan. Experiment with different flavors, ingredients, and recipes to find your favorite desserts that fit your dietary needs and taste preferences. With a little creativity and planning, you can indulge in delicious treats without compromising your health, one bite at a time.

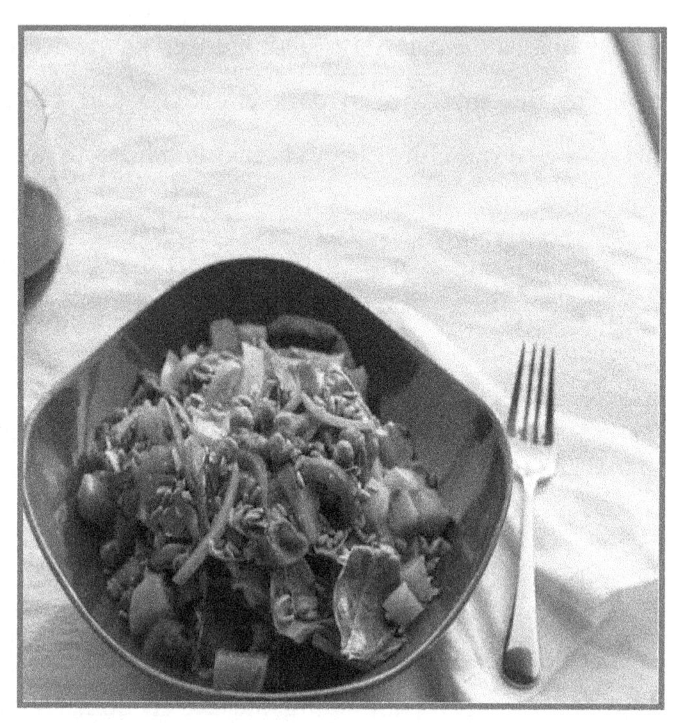

CHAPTER EIGHT

Comforting Casseroles for Cozy Evenings

Nothing is more satisfying on a cold night than a hot and full dish of casserole. The smell of melted cheese, meat and vegetables bubbling in the kitchen makes it comfortable and happy. Locating comforting dishes that also help maintain blood sugar can be difficult for people living with diabetes. In this chapter, we will cover some casseroles which are specially made to cater for diabetics' needs without having to compromise on taste.

Chicken and Vegetable Quinoa Casserole:
This healthy casserole is filled with proteins, fibers, and vital nutrients making it ideal for individuals controlling their diabetic conditions. Start cooking quinoa as per the instructions given on its packet; then stir in cooked chicken breast, sautéed vegetables such as onions, bell peppers, zucchini

among others and mix all together using Greek yogurt based creamy sauce along with the herbs of your choice. Finally, add some grated cheese on top before baking until golden brown and bubbly. You can serve this warming casserole alongside a salad as a complete meal that guarantees satisfaction from the inside.

Beef and Mushroom Cauliflower Rice Casserole

In this low-carb casserole, swap traditional rice for cauliflower rice, which has a wealth of taste and texture. Brown lean ground beef with onions, garlic, and mushrooms until it is done and smells nicely. Include cauliflower rice, diced tomatoes, tomato sauce and Italian herbs in the mixture then pour it into a baking dish and top with some shredded cheese. Bake until the cheese melts and becomes bubbly; you may choose to garnish with fresh parsley or basil to serve for colour or freshness if desired. On cold nights spent with family members this comforting casserole is perfect.

Spinach and Artichoke Chicken Casserole:

A rich creamy spinach dip and artichoke casserole comes in handy when you feel like having something hearty. Start by sautéing chicken breast until golden brown on both sides but fully cooked through, mix in cooked spinach, artichoke hearts Greek yogurt cream cheese grated Parmesan cheese.Transfer to baking dish sprinkle mozzarella cheese over.Bake until cheese is melted bubbly,pair this indulgent casserole with roasted vegetables or crispy green salad as a delicious balanced meal.

Turkey and Sweet Potato Shepherd's Pie

This tasty variation of a traditional shepherd's pie is rich in lean protein, complex carbohydrates and colorful veggies. Brown the turkey with onions, carrots and celery until it is cooked through and aromatic; then transfer this to a baking dish. Cover it with mashed sweet potatoes that have been given a little bit of nutmeg and cinnamon flavorings, then bake at 350°F for about half an hour or until golden brown on top. Serve this delicious hotpot alongside some boiled green beans or roasted Brussels sprouts for a warm, well-balanced meal perfect for sharing with family.

Tuna and Broccoli Casserole with Cauliflower Cream Sauce:

Relish the flavors of tuna casserole without the high fat content and refined carbs by using cauliflower cream sauce. Steam cauliflower until tender, then blend it with low-fat milk, garlic, and nutritional yeast until smooth and creamy. Mix cooked tuna, steamed broccoli florets, and cooked whole-grain pasta in a baking dish, then pour the cauliflower cream sauce over the top. Bake until heated through and bubbly, then garnish with a sprinkle of breadcrumbs for added crunch This lighter dish will satisfy your craving for comfort food without deviating from your diabetes control plan.

Mediterranean Eggplant and Lentil Casserole

This full flavored and healthy eggplant and lentil casserole will make your palate long for the

Mediterranean. First, sauté diced aubergines, onions and garlic until golden brown and tender; then add cooked lentils, chopped tomatoes, olives, dried oregano and basil. Pour the mixture into a baking dish before crumbling on top some feta cheese. Put in the oven till it becomes heated through and bubbly then serve this filling casserole with whole grain bread on the side or a crispy garden salad as a complete meal full of Mediterranean flavors.

Mexican Chicken and Cauliflower Rice Casserole

If you are tired of monotonous suppers, try this zesty Mexican style chicken beefed up with cauliflower rice in a casserole. Sear chicken breast together with onions, garlic cloves and bell peppers until fully cooked over medium heat; next mix with cauliflower rice (grated cauliflower), black beans, corn kernels, tomatoes dices seasoned in Mexican spices like cumin, chili powder or paprika. Strew shredded cheese over it before baking to melt the cheese while top is bubbly golden brown; enjoy this lively casserole by at least greek yoghurt spoonfuls alongside lime squeezed for freshness sake.

Cheesy Broccoli and Quinoa Casserole

This comforting casserole is packed with nutrient-rich ingredients such as quinoa, broccoli, and cheese, making it a perfect choice for individuals managing diabetes. Cook quinoa according to package instructions, then mix it with steamed broccoli florets, Greek yogurt, shredded cheddar cheese, and a touch of Dijon mustard for added flavor. Transfer the mixture to a baking dish and top with a sprinkle of breadcrumbs for added crunch. Bake until heated through and bubbly, then serve this satisfying casserole with a side of roasted vegetables or a crisp green salad for a balanced and delicious meal.

Italian Sausage and Pepper Cauliflower Rice Casserole

Savor the robust tastes of Italian cooking with this gratifying and flavorful casserole of sausage and pepper cauliflower rice. Brown Italian sausage with onions, garlic, and bell peppers until cooked through and fragrant, then mix in cauliflower rice, diced tomatoes, tomato sauce, and Italian herbs such as oregano, basil, and thyme. Transfer the mixture to a baking dish and top with a layer of shredded mozzarella cheese. Bake until the cheese is melted and bubbly, then serve this flavorful casserole with a sprinkle of chopped parsley for a pop of color and freshness.

Veggie and Bean Enchilada Casserole

Enjoy the robust tastes of Tex-Mex cuisine with this filling and healthy bean and vegetable enchilada dish.. Layer corn tortillas with cooked black beans, sautéed vegetables such as bell peppers, onions, and zucchini, and a tangy enchilada sauce made with diced tomatoes, green chilies, and Mexican spices. Top with a sprinkle of shredded cheese and bake until heated through and bubbly. Serve this vibrant casserole with a dollop of Greek yogurt or a squeeze of lime juice for a burst of freshness and flavor.

Casseroles offer a comforting and convenient way to enjoy delicious and nutritious meals while managing diabetes effectively. By including wholesome ingredients such as lean proteins, vibrant vegetables, and whole grains, you can create hearty and satisfying dishes that support blood sugar control and promote overall health and well-being. Experiment with different flavors, ingredients, and recipes to find your favorite comforting casseroles that fit your dietary needs and taste preferences. With a little creativity and planning, you can indulge in cozy evenings filled with delicious food and warm memories, one casserole at a time.

CHAPTER NINE

Flavorful Salads for Vibrant Meals

Salads are often viewed as a mundane or uninspired meal option, but they have the potential to be so much more. With the right combination of fresh ingredients, flavorful dressings, and creative toppings, salads can transform into vibrant and satisfying meals that excite the taste buds and nourish the body. In this chapter, we'll explore a variety of flavorful salad recipes specifically tailored to meet the needs of individuals managing diabetes, providing both delicious flavors and essential nutrients to support overall health and well-being.

Grilled Chicken Caesar Salad

Upgrade the traditional Caesar salad by adding succulent grilled chicken breast for a filling, high-protein lunch that works well for any time of day.. Start by marinating chicken breasts in a mixture of olive oil, lemon juice, garlic, and Italian herbs, then grill until cooked through and lightly charred. Arrange crisp romaine lettuce leaves on a plate and top with slices of grilled chicken, shaved Parmesan cheese, and whole-grain croutons. Drizzle with a homemade Caesar dressing made with Greek yogurt, anchovies, Dijon mustard, and lemon juice for a lighter and healthier twist on a beloved classic.

Quinoa and Black Bean Fiesta Salad

This colorful, flavorful, and nutrient-rich quinoa and black bean fiesta salad is perfect for celebrating the flavors of Latin cooking. Cook quinoa according to package instructions and let it cool, then mix it with cooked black beans, diced bell peppers, corn kernels, cherry tomatoes, and chopped cilantro. Toss with a zesty lime vinaigrette made with olive oil, lime juice, garlic, and cumin for added flavor. Serve this festive salad as a stand alone meal or as a flavorful side dish to grilled chicken or fish for a satisfying and nutritious meal option.

Mediterranean Chickpea and Feta Salad

This tasty, refreshing chickpea and feta salad will take your taste buds to the sunny shores of the Mediterranean. It's a great dish to serve throughout the warmer months.. Mix canned chickpeas with diced cucumbers, cherry tomatoes, red onions, Kalamata olives, and crumbled feta cheese in a large bowl. Drizzle with a tangy vinaigrette made with olive oil, red wine vinegar, lemon juice, garlic, and oregano for added brightness and flavor. Serve this vibrant salad as a standalone meal or as a delicious side dish to grilled lamb or chicken souvlaki for a taste of the Mediterranean at home.

Asian-Inspired Sesame Ginger Tofu Salad:

Satisfy your cravings for Asian flavors with this vibrant and protein-packed sesame ginger tofu salad that's bursting with freshness and flavor. Start by marinating extra-firm tofu in a mixture of soy sauce, sesame oil, ginger, and garlic, then bake until golden brown and crispy. Toss crisp mixed greens with shredded carrots, sliced cucumbers, red cabbage, and chopped scallions in a large bowl. Top with slices of baked tofu and drizzle with a homemade sesame ginger dressing made with rice vinegar, sesame oil, honey, and grated ginger for a delicious and satisfying salad that's perfect for lunch or dinner.

Berry and Goat Cheese Spinach Salad:
Savor the sweet and savory tastes of this delicious spinach salad with berries and goat cheese, ideal for summer eating.. Toss fresh baby spinach leaves with sliced strawberries, blueberries, raspberries, and crumbled goat cheese in a large bowl. Drizzle with a tangy balsamic vinaigrette made with olive oil, balsamic vinegar, honey, and Dijon mustard for added flavor. Top with toasted pecans or walnuts for added crunch and texture. Serve this refreshing salad as a standalone meal or as a delicious side dish to grilled chicken or salmon for a light and flavorful summer meal.

Thai-Inspired Peanut Chicken Salad:

This vivid and tasty peanut chicken salad, inspired by Thai cuisine, will transport your taste senses to the busy streets of Bangkok and satisfy your demands for strong and exotic flavors. Start by marinating chicken breast in a mixture of soy sauce, lime juice, garlic, and ginger, then grill until cooked through and lightly charred. Toss crisp mixed greens with shredded cabbage, julienne carrots, sliced bell peppers, and chopped cilantro in a large bowl. Top with slices of grilled chicken and drizzle with a creamy peanut dressing made with peanut butter, coconut milk, lime juice, soy sauce, and chili paste for a delicious and satisfying salad that's perfect for any occasion.

Roasted Vegetable and Quinoa Salad with Lemon Tahini Dressing:

Enjoy the earthy flavors of roasted vegetables paired with nutty quinoa and creamy tahini dressing in this hearty and nutritious salad that's perfect for cooler weather dining. Roast a variety of vegetables such as sweet potatoes, carrots, cauliflower, and Brussels sprouts until caramelized and tender, then let them cool. Mix the roasted vegetables with cooked quinoa, chopped parsley, and toasted almonds or pine nuts in a large bowl. Drizzle with a tangy lemon tahini dressing made with tahini, lemon juice, garlic, and olive oil for added richness and flavor. Serve this hearty salad as a standalone meal or as a delicious side dish to grilled meats or fish for a satisfying and nutritious meal option.

Caprese Salad with Balsamic Glaze:

Savor the flavors of this traditional Caprese salad, which are straightforward yet sophisticated. For extra depth and richness, sprinkle some tangy balsamic sauce over it.. Put some fresh mozzarella cheese, juicy tomato slices, and basil leaves on a dish. Drizzle with some balsamic sauce and season with flaky sea salt and freshly ground black pepper. Serve this refreshing salad as a starter to a meal or as a light and satisfying lunch option that's bursting with flavor and freshness.

Shrimp and Avocado Cobb Salad:

Treat yourself to a delicious and protein-packed shrimp and avocado Cobb salad that's perfect for satisfying your hunger and fueling your body with essential nutrients. Arrange crisp mixed greens on a platter and top with cooked shrimp, sliced hard-boiled eggs, diced avocado, crumbled bacon, cherry tomatoes, and crumbled blue cheese. Drizzle with a tangy ranch dressing made with Greek yogurt, buttermilk, garlic, and fresh herbs for added flavor. Serve this hearty salad as a stand alone meal or as a satisfying side dish to grilled chicken or steak for a delicious and nutritious meal option.

Warm Lentil and Roasted Vegetable Salad:

Warm lentil and roasted vegetable salad is a filling and substantial dish that is ideal for dining outside in the cooler months. Roast a variety of vegetables such as carrots, parsnips, beets, and red onions until caramelized and tender, then let them cool slightly. Mix the roasted vegetables with cooked lentils, chopped parsley, and crumbled feta cheese in a large bowl. Drizzle with a tangy vinaigrette made with red wine vinegar, Dijon mustard, garlic, and olive oil for added brightness and flavor. Serve this satisfying salad as a standalone meal or as a delicious side dish to grilled sausages or roasted chicken for a comforting and nutritious meal option.

Salads offer a versatile and delicious way to enjoy nutritious and flavorful meals while managing diabetes effectively. By incorporating a variety of fresh ingredients, vibrant flavors, and creative dressings, you can create salads that excite the taste buds and nourish the body. Experiment with different combinations of fruits, vegetables, proteins, and dressings to find your favorite salad recipes that fit your dietary needs and taste preferences. With a little creativity and planning, you can enjoy vibrant and satisfying meals that support your health and well-being on your journey to better diabetes management.

CHAPTER TEN

Meal Planning and Prepping for Success

Being diagnosed with diabetes can be overwhelming, but it's also an opportunity to take control of your health through mindful meal planning and preparation. By making informed choices about what you eat and how you prepare your meals, you can effectively manage your blood sugar levels and improve your overall well-being. In this guide, we'll explore the importance of meal planning and prepping for success in diabetes management, providing practical tips and strategies to help you navigate this journey with confidence and ease.

Understanding the Importance of Meal Planning:

Meal planning is a crucial aspect of managing diabetes, as it allows you to make thoughtful decisions about the foods you eat and their impact on your blood sugar levels. By planning your meals in advance, you can ensure that you're consuming a balanced diet that includes a variety of nutrient-rich foods such as fruits, vegetables, whole grains, lean proteins, and healthy fats. Additionally, meal planning can help you avoid impulsive food choices and overeating, both of which can lead to spikes in blood sugar levels and other complications associated with diabetes.

Benefits of Meal Planning:

Blood Sugar Control: Planning your meals allows you to choose foods that won't cause rapid spikes or drops in blood sugar levels, helping you maintain stable energy levels throughout the day.

Weight Management: Meal planning can help you control portion sizes and make healthier food choices, which can contribute to weight loss or maintenance, an important aspect of diabetes management.

Time and Cost Savings: By planning your meals in advance, you can streamline your grocery shopping and cooking processes, saving both time and money in the long run.

Improved Nutrient Intake: Meal planning encourages you to include a variety of nutrient-rich foods in your diet, ensuring that you're getting all the essential vitamins, minerals, and antioxidants your body needs to function optimally.

Tips for Successful Meal Planning and Prepping:

Set Realistic Goals: Start by setting realistic and achievable goals for your meal planning efforts. Consider factors such as your schedule, dietary preferences, and nutritional needs when creating your meal plans.

Create a Weekly Meal Plan: Dedicate some time each week to plan out your meals and snacks for the upcoming week. Consider incorporating a variety of flavors, textures, and cuisines to keep your meals exciting and satisfying.

Focus on Balance: Aim to include a balance of carbohydrates, proteins, and fats in each meal to help stabilize your blood sugar levels and promote feelings of fullness and satisfaction.

Choose Whole Foods: Opt for whole, minimally processed foods whenever possible, as they tend to be higher in nutrients and lower in added sugars and unhealthy fats. Fill your plate with plenty of fruits, vegetables, whole grains, lean proteins, and healthy fats to support your overall health and well-being.

Batch Cooking: Consider batch cooking large quantities of staple foods such as grains, beans, and proteins at the beginning of the week to streamline your meal preparation process. Divide the cooked ingredients into portion-sized containers and store them in the refrigerator or freezer for easy grab-and-go meals throughout the week.

Prep Ahead: Spend some time each week washing, chopping, and portioning out fruits, vegetables, and other ingredients to make meal preparation faster and more efficient. Having prepped ingredients on hand makes it easier to throw together quick and nutritious meals, even on busy days.

Use Smart Cooking Techniques: Experiment with cooking techniques such as roasting, grilling, steaming, and sautéing to enhance the flavor and texture of your meals without relying on excess fats or sugars. Get creative with herbs, spices, and condiments to add depth and complexity to your dishes.

Portion Control: Pay attention to portion sizes and serving sizes to avoid overeating and unnecessary calorie intake. Use measuring cups, spoons, and kitchen scales to portion out foods accurately, especially when it comes to carbohydrate-rich foods like grains, fruits, and starchy vegetables.

Stay Flexible: Be willing to adapt your meal plans and recipes based on changes in your schedule, preferences, or dietary needs. Flexibility is key to long-term success in meal planning and prepping, so don't be afraid to experiment and try new things.

Sample Meal Plan:

Here's a sample meal plan to help you get started on your journey to successful meal planning and prepping:

Breakfast:

Greek yogurt parfait with mixed berries and granola

Whole-grain toast with avocado and sliced tomatoes

Scrambled eggs with spinach, bell peppers, and feta cheese

Lunch:

Quinoa salad with roasted vegetables and grilled chicken

Turkey and avocado wrap with whole-grain tortilla

Lentil soup with side salad and whole-grain roll

Dinner:

Baked salmon served with steamed broccoli and roasted sweet potatoes

Vegetable stir-fry with tofu and brown rice

Turkey chili with mixed greens salad and whole-grain cornbread

Snacks:

Sliced apple with almond butter

Carrot sticks with hummus

Greek yogurt with mixed nuts and berries

Meal planning and prepping are essential tools for successfully managing diabetes and promoting overall health and well-being. By taking the time to plan out your meals, choose nutrient-rich foods, and prepare ahead of time, you can ensure that you're making informed choices that support your blood sugar control and long-term health goals. Remember to stay flexible, experiment with new recipes and ingredients, and listen to your body's hunger and fullness cues as you navigate this journey. You may savor tasty and nourishing meals that feed your body and soul, one bite at a time, with commitment, awareness, and a little preparation.

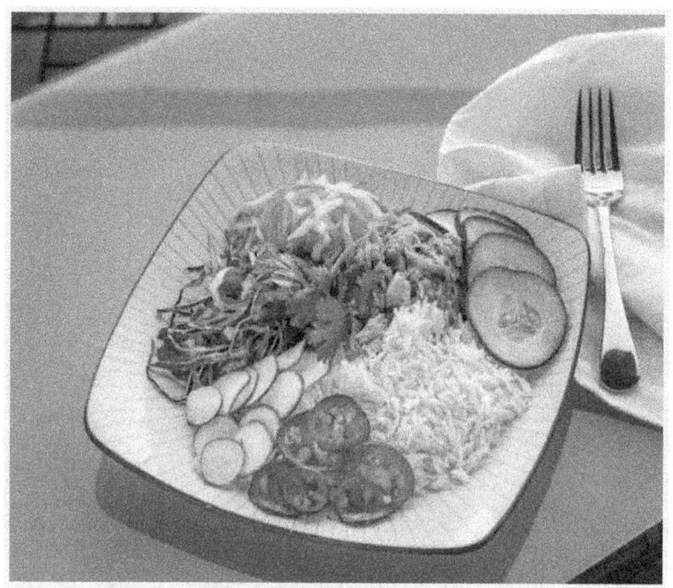

CHAPTER ELEVEN

Staying Motivated and Positive on Your Diabetic Journey

Being newly diagnosed with diabetes can be a challenging and overwhelming experience. It's normal to feel a range of emotions, including fear, frustration, and uncertainty about what the future holds. However, it's important to remember that living with diabetes is not a life sentence, but rather an opportunity to take control of your health and well-being. In this guide, we'll explore practical tips and strategies for staying motivated and positive on your diabetic journey, empowering you to navigate this path with resilience, optimism, and confidence.

Educate Yourself:

One of the most empowering things you can do after being diagnosed with diabetes is to educate yourself about the condition. Take the time to learn about the different types of diabetes, how it affects the body, and the role of diet, exercise, medication, and monitoring in managing the condition. Knowledge is power, and the more you understand about diabetes, the better equipped you'll be to make informed decisions about your health and well-being.

Set Realistic Goals:

Setting realistic and achievable goals is essential for staying motivated and making progress on your diabetic journey. Start by identifying specific areas of your health and lifestyle that you'd like to improve, whether it's managing your blood sugar levels, losing weight, increasing physical activity, or adopting healthier eating habits. Break down your goals into smaller, actionable steps, and celebrate your progress along the way. Remember that change takes time, so be patient with yourself and focus on making gradual and sustainable improvements.

Surround Yourself with Support:

Navigating the challenges of diabetes can be easier when you have a strong support system in place.

Surround yourself with family members, friends, healthcare professionals, and others who understand and support your journey. Lean on them for encouragement, guidance, and practical assistance when needed. Consider joining a diabetes support group or online community where you can connect with others who are going through similar experiences and share tips, advice, and encouragement.

Practice Self-Care:

Taking care of yourself physically, mentally, and emotionally is crucial for managing diabetes and maintaining a positive outlook on life. Make self-care a priority by prioritizing adequate sleep, engaging in regular physical activity, managing stress through relaxation techniques such as deep breathing, meditation, or yoga, and indulging in activities that bring you joy and fulfillment. Remember that self-care looks different for everyone, so find what works best for you and make it a regular part of your routine.

Focus on the Positives:

While living with diabetes comes with its challenges, it's important to focus on the positives and acknowledge the strengths and resilience that you possess. Instead of dwelling on what you can't eat or do, focus on what you can do to take control of your health and live your best life. Celebrate your victories, no matter how small, and recognize the progress you're making towards your goals. Cultivate an attitude of gratitude and find joy in the little things that bring happiness and fulfillment to your life.

Stay Flexible and Adapt:

Living with diabetes requires flexibility and adaptability, as your body's needs and circumstances may change over time. Be open to trying new foods, recipes, and lifestyle changes to see what works best for you and your diabetes management. If you experience setbacks or challenges along the way, don't be discouraged.

Instead, view them as opportunities for growth and learning, and use them as motivation to keep moving forward towards your goals.

Celebrate Your Successes:
Take the time to celebrate your successes, no matter how small, and acknowledge the progress you've made on your diabetic journey. Whether it's achieving a target blood sugar level, sticking to a healthy eating plan, or reaching a milestone in your fitness journey, celebrate your accomplishments and give yourself credit for your hard work and dedication. Treat yourself to something special, whether it's a relaxing day at the spa, a favorite meal, or a fun activity with loved ones, to reward yourself for your efforts and keep your motivation high.

Stay Connected with Healthcare Professionals:
Regular communication and follow-up with your healthcare team are essential for managing diabetes effectively and staying on track with your treatment

plan. Schedule regular check-ups with your doctor, diabetes educator, nutritionist, and other healthcare professionals to monitor your progress, address any concerns or questions you may have, and make adjustments to your treatment plan as needed. Don't hesitate to reach out for support or guidance whenever you need it, as your healthcare team is there to help you every step of the way.

Practice Mindfulness and Resilience:
Cultivating mindfulness and resilience can help you cope with the challenges and uncertainties of living with diabetes and maintain a positive outlook on life. Practice mindfulness techniques such as deep breathing, meditation, or visualization to stay grounded and present in the moment, even during stressful or difficult times. Cultivate resilience by reframing negative thoughts and setbacks into opportunities for growth and learning, and by maintaining a sense of optimism and hope for the future.

Find Purpose and Meaning:

Living with diabetes can be an opportunity to find purpose and meaning in your life by taking control of your health and well-being and making a positive impact on yourself and others. Find activities, hobbies, or causes that bring you joy and fulfillment, whether it's volunteering, pursuing a passion project, or spending time with loved ones. Focus on what truly matters to you and what gives your life meaning, and let that guide you on your diabetic journey towards health, happiness, and fulfillment.

Living with diabetes is a journey that comes with its challenges, but it's also an opportunity to take control of your health, embrace resilience, and cultivate a positive outlook on life. By educating yourself, setting realistic goals, surrounding yourself with support, practicing self-care, focusing on the positives, staying flexible and adaptable, celebrating your successes, staying connected with healthcare professionals, practicing mindfulness and resilience, and finding purpose and meaning, you can navigate your diabetic journey with confidence, optimism, and resilience. Remember that you're not alone on this journey, and that with determination, perseverance, and a positive mindset, you can overcome any obstacles and thrive in spite of diabetes.

CONCLUSION

Starting a diabetic journey can be daunting, but armed with knowledge, support, and a positive mindset, it becomes a path filled with opportunities for growth, resilience, and empowerment. Throughout this guide, we've explored the importance of meal planning and preparation, staying motivated and positive, and embracing self-care and mindfulness on your diabetic journey.

As you navigate the twists and turns of life with diabetes, remember that you are not alone. Lean on your support system, whether it's friends, family, or healthcare professionals, for guidance, encouragement, and understanding. Embrace the power of education and empowerment, taking charge of your health through informed decisions and proactive management strategies.

No matter how tiny your victory may be, realize the strides you've achieved and celebrate them. Stay flexible and adaptable, willing to try new things and adjust your approach as needed. Cultivate resilience and mindfulness, finding strength and peace in the present moment, even amidst life's challenges.

Above all, remember that living with diabetes is not a limitation, but rather an invitation to live your best life with vitality, purpose, and joy. Accept your diabetic journey with confidence and optimism, knowing that with dedication, determination, and a positive attitude, you can thrive in spite of diabetes and live a life filled with health, happiness, and fulfillment.

www.ingramcontent.com/pod-product-compliance
Lightning Source LLC
Chambersburg PA
CBHW072337270726
48659CB00022B/1781